Contents

Balancing on one foot 1

Jenga 2

Pennies game 3

Balancing relay 4

Simon Says 5

Breathing exercise 9

Take a walk in nature 10

Bell exercise 11

Breathing companion 12

Sense of smell 13

Read your heartbeat 14

Positive mission statement 15

Embrace every feeling 16

Create a mind jar 17

Body scan 19

Visualization.. 20

Yoga 21

Practice gratitude 22

Hand tracing.. 23

Stay calm and composed.................................... 24

Blind man 25

Balloons off the ground 26

What's in the bag? 27

Blindfolded taste test 28

Balance beam 29

Listening game.. 31

Pitching pennies 32

In and out hangman.. 33

Pen and pencil games 35

Sock toss 37

Indoor obstacle course 38

Puzzles 39

Card games 40

Build a fort 41

Dominoes 43

Marshmallow tinker toys 44

Make your own story 45

DIY catapult 46

Ice tower excavation 47

Balancing on one foot

Purpose: Body awareness, Focus, Awareness, Mindful seeing

Best For: Ages 3+, groups or one-on-one

What you need: Nothing

This is a simple game to develop focus and body awareness. It can be used to combat boredom while standing in a line, for example.

Ask your child to focus her gaze on a point slightly below eye level. Then ask her to stand on one leg and keep her gaze on the focal point. How long can she balance like this?

Try the other leg. To make it more difficult, engage your child in conversation. Ask her to sing something or to balance with her eyes closed. With a group of kids, you can see who can balance the longest time.

Jenga

Purpose: Body awareness, Focus, Awareness, Understanding emotions

Best For: Ages 6+, one-on-one

What you need: Jenga the game

Jenga isn't just for kids–it's a lot of fun for everyone. It teaches you how to pay attention, too. You can make it mindful by asking your child to pay attention to whatever it is that distracts her from the game.

Is she able to notice what made her lose focus?

Did thoughts or emotions make her lose concentration?

How about if you ask her tough questions as you play?

Pennies game

Purpose: Detail Awareness, Focus, Awareness

Best For: Ages 3+, groups or one-on-one

What you need: One penny for each player, a basket

Everyone gets a penny and a minute to study it in detail. The pennies are then placed back in the basket. Each player has to pick their penny out of all the pennies and say how they knew it was theirs. This game can be played with different objects.

Balancing relay

Purpose: Body awareness, Focus, Awareness

Best For: Ages 5+, groups or one-on-one

What you need: A spoon and some water (or a spoon and a potato) per team

Similar to the egg-and-spoon race, this game teaches both focus and body awareness. The idea is to carry a spoon full of water to the next kid without spilling a drop. You can make it into a relay race if you are playing with a group of kids. To take it to the next level, ask your child to walk backwards or sideways while balancing the spoon.

Simon Says

Purpose: Mindful listening and seeing, Focus, Awareness

Best For: Ages 4+, groups or one-on-one

What you need: Room to move

The classic Simon Says game uses both mindful seeing and listening skills. When the leader (the designated Simon) issues her command verbally and shows what to do visually, kids are challenged to pay attention to both visual and auditory input and discern whether or not to act.

The clue is that there's a conflict between what they see visually and what they are instructed to do verbally.

Remember, you are only allowed to act when the leader says "Simon says" before the instruction.

We tend to act without thinking, and this game demonstrates just that.

Simon Says is a fun way to practice mindfulness by paying attention to outer experiences.

Here's how the game works.

Choose who will take the role of Simon. It's best if you model first. Next, Simon stands in front of the player(s) and issues instructions for physical actions and shows how to do them.

The instructions should be followed only if prefaced with the phrase "Simon says".

Players win when they follow an instruction that is preceded by the phrase "Simon says".

Players fail if they perform the action without the "Simon says" phrase or if they fail to perform the action when the phrase "Simon says" is used before the instruction.

If you want keep the game less competitive, you don't have to eliminate players when they fail.

When you play with just one child, you can decide to switch roles when the player fails three times.

It doesn't matter if you can actually perform the physical tasks, an attempt is enough. The ability to distinguish fake commands is what matters in this fun game.

Here are some amusing examples:

Simon says play air guitar. Simon demonstrates playing air guitar.

Simons says waddle like a penguin. Simon does a penguin impression.

Simon says cry like a baby. Simon cries like a baby.

Simon says tickle your feet. Simon tickles his feet.

Simon says giggle. Simon giggles.

Simon says freeze. Simon freezes.

Simon says spin around once. Simon spins around.

Simon says spin around twice. Simon spins around twice.

Spin around three times. Simon spins around thrice.

Did you attempt to spin around after this last command?

If you spun around, you failed. Simon didn't say "Simon says" before the command

When you are done playing, talk about the experience. Ask your child if it was hard or easy to pay attention to the instructions. Was it hard to pay attention to the instructions when they were excited and having fun?

Discuss how paying attention to what we see and hear could be helpful.

Breathing exercise

Breathing exercises help in relaxing and training the mind to be calm and balanced, regardless of the circumstances.

How to:

- Get the child to sit in a calm environment, in a comfortable position.

- Ask the child to breathe normally and to observe their breath.

- After a couple of minutes, ask them to take a deep breath and once again observe the inhaling and exhaling procedure.

- Repeat this activity at least 5 to 10 times every day.

Take a walk in nature

A walk in a natural setting such as a forest or a park makes one more aware and vigilant of their surroundings. Mindfulness activities are about making oneself more attentive, and this activity will help you achieve just that.

How to:

- Choose a garden, trek, or any outdoor area with greenery.

- Stock up on healthy snacks and water to stay hydrated.

- Let the child walk around in a relaxed manner. Ask them to observe everything they find on their trail and listen to the sounds of the birds, the wind, and the stream if there is one.

- This mindful walk will awaken all their senses and connect them with nature.

Bell exercise

Tis fun exercise will make the child relate to the present moment and enhance their auditory senses. This can be an individual activity or a group activity. You will need a medium or large-sized bell and a noise-free room.

How to:

- Make the child sit in a hquiet place. If it is a group of children, ask them to sit in a circle.

- Now ring a bell and ask the kids to pay attention to the sound of the bell, and the vibrations it generates.

- Ask them to remain silent, and when they stop hearing the sound of the bell, ask them to raise their hand.

- Let them stay silent for a minute more to pay attention to the other sounds they can hear around them.

- Finally, ask the children to describe their hearing experiences before and after the bell was rung.

Breathing companion

In this mindfulness activity, children will use a soft toy as a breathing companion, which will engage them and also help them understand how breathing can affect the vibrations in their body.

How to:

- Place a soft or a stuffed toy on the child's stomach.
- Now ask the child to breathe normally and observe the movement of their breathing companion.
- Next, ask them to breathe heavily and observe how their companion moves.
- Repeat the same while breathing slowly.
- They will notice that their breathing companion falls when they breathe heavily and stays intact when they breathe normally or slowly.
- This activity can be used to teach kids about the importance of maintaining a balanced mindset in all situations in life.

Sense of smell

This is a simple yet powerful activity to train kids on exercising their sense of smell and how it can have an impact on improving their mindfulness. Soothing aromas can sometimes relieve anxiety and stress too.

How to:

- Place various objects with distinct smells in front of the child.

- Ask them to pick each item, smell it, and then describe it.

- When they smell, ask them to close their eyes and focus all their attention on the smell alone.

- Choose objects with appealing fragrances so that at the end of the activity, they experience a feeling of freshness.

Read your heartbeat

This is a regular jumping exercise but with a twist – you have to read your heartbeat when you do.

How to:

- Ask the kids to stand still and observe their heartbeat.

- Now make them jump continuously for a minute or so, without any interruption.

- Ask them to pay attention to their heartbeat now.

- At the end of this fun activity, ask them to record their observations.

Positive mission statement

Use this activity to reinforce a positive attitude and motivation, which can play a critical role in improving mindfulness.

How to:

- Ask the children to sit in a relaxed position, with a calm mind.
- Ask them to take a couple of deep breaths, close their eyes, and think about their lives and what inspires them.
- Next, give them 15 minutes to come up with a positive slogan or mission for their lives.
- This positive mission statement can be practiced by them regularly to reinforce the zeal and confidence in their everyday lives.

Embrace every feeling

Feelings are just feelings, and they are temporary. It is essential for children to learn that there is no good feeling or bad feeling, and this activity helps them with that.

How to:

- Ask the child to think about two past experiences: a happy one and a sad one.

- Now ask them to describe both the instances in detail.

- When they are done with the explanation, ask how it feels in the present moment, and if those feelings matter to them in the current moment.

- When they talk about it, they will realize how liberating it is to let go off irrelevant thoughts about what happened in the past.

Create a mind jar

Although rare, just doing nothing and fidgeting around with things can sometimes help in relieving tense muscles. And if the things around are really nice and colorful, it is all the better.

How to:

- Take a clear jar with a tight lid to secure it properly.

- Help your child add hot water to the jar until it fills up to the 3/4th mark.

- Now, it's time to have fun with glitter. You can stick to one color or go crazy with as many as you want.

- Let it sit for some time and secure the lid with hot glue so that it won't spill over later.

- That's it! Your very own mind jar is ready! Shake the jar and see the colorful glitter dance for you.

You may use this mind jar, every time you feel stuck with thoughts or even when you are stressed.

Tip: A parent or guardian must supervise children during this activity. Parents are advised to be very careful while using hot water or hot glue so that children do not harm themselves.

Body scan

This is a simple but thoroughly relaxing activity that helps in developing a mindful and attentive personality. The ideal time for this activity is before your child's bedtime, as it can help them relax and sleep soundly.

How to:

- Make the child sit in a relaxed position.

- Ask them to take a couple of deep breaths.

- Now ask them to lie down comfortably and close their eyes.

- Ask them to focus on each little part of the body, starting from head to toe, as they inhale and exhale. They must move their attention from the tip of their toe to feet, then legs and slowly upwards to the head.

- To end this activity, they must once again spend a few minutes running their attention throughout the body.

Visualization

Guided imagery or visualization for kids is an engaging activity. The visualization you choose may vary from short and simple to quite deep.

How to:

- Choose a topic which suits the child or kids in one group, and something that will also address their concerns. For instance, you can pick a motivational topic before a test or competition.
- Ask children to sit in a relaxed and comfortable posture and close their eyes.
- Give them specific and clear instructions, right from the beginning of the visualization process to the end.
- To make the activity very soothing, you may also choose to play music such as nature sounds or calming rhythmic playlists

Yoga

Yoga has enormous benefits, not just for the body but also for the mind. It helps in improving focus and concentration levels too.

How to:

- Start with basic yoga exercises while explaining children about the benefits of each of them.
- Yoga, introduced at an early age in life, helps a child in building self-esteem, physical and mental awareness.

Practice gratitude

Being thankful and expressing gratitude plays a pivotal role in becoming a better human. For every little blessing or favor we receive from anyone, we must be grateful.

How to:

- Kids can practice gratitude by thanking their parents for providing them with food, shelter, and a good life.
- They may also express gratitude to their teachers, friends, and elders.
- They can express this aloud or write it down in a journal.

Hand tracing

Who knew that an activity as simple as tracing your hand could also contribute to mindfulness?

How to:

- Ask the child to take a blank paper and place their non-writing hand on it first.

- Let them start tracing, using the other hand, on a sheet of paper. This would be the easy part.

- Now ask them to place their writing hand on the paper and trace it with the non-writing hand.

- Ask them how it feels? Not very easy, but that's the trick, to challenge your mind to perform non-routine activities with ease. This will prove beneficial in training the mind in doing various activities with ease.

Stay calm and composed

It is easier said than done! No matter how much one may try, it is quite natural for anyone to lose their mind when things are not going right. But with a little patience, you can slowly train your child to take little steps towards having a calm or balanced reaction to any unforeseen event or situation in life.

How to:

- Every time something agitates them, ask them to try something like drinking water, counting numbers, taking a deep breath, or going for a walk to calm or distract themselves.
- These small steps will bring a significant change if practiced consistently.

Blind man

We all love playing the blindfold game, but do you know that it can offer plenty of mindfulness benefits too?

How to:

- Choose one kid to be a blind man and blindfold him/her.

- Now the blind man has to hear the sounds and observe the sensations around, to identify others who are playing together.

- The blind man has to catch as many people as possible.

- The challenge here is to win at the game when the most important sensory organ; your vision is not supporting you.

Balloons off the ground

This is one such game which can be enjoyed by not just kids but elders, pets, and everyone else too. The game compels the participants to focus and improves mindfulness also.

How to:

- Get a few colorful balloons.
- Ask the kids to blow the balloon as big as they can, under the supervision of a parent.
- Now the challenge is to play with the balloon and keep it up in the air.
- They lose a point every time the balloon touches the ground.

What's in the bag?

What's in the bag is a fun game for young children; it can be used as an educational tool too.

How to:

- Place random items of various shapes, sizes, and textures in a bag.

- Ask the child to reach into the bag using just one hand and identify the item without looking at it. You may even blindfold them to make it more challenging and activate their sense of touch.

- The challenge in mindfulness game lies in trying to name the objects correctly, the more, the better. Having a timer would make it more fun.

Blindfolded taste test

Awareness of each of the sensory organs also plays a crucial role in developing mindfulness in kids and adults. A blindfolded taste test is a game to activate or test your taste buds. Here's how it's done.

How to:

- Blindfold any one player.
- Place any ten random food items such as sauces, cookies, chocolate, juices, fruits, etc., on a table.
- Now the other players have to make the blindfolded player taste each food item.
- The blindfolded player has to guess the name of each item.
- The player who identifies the most number of food items wins the game.

Tip: Do not include any allergens or food items such as nuts, dairy, gluten, etc., that children could be allergic to.

Balance beam

Balancing beam is easier to set up than you think. All you need is some colored sticky tape, and you're good to play for hours.

You will need:

- Colored mask tape (multiple colors for more fun)
- Space to play

How to:

- Clear some space in a room and clean the floor.
- Stick the length of the tape to create straight or curved lines to walk on.
- You can use multiple colors and have unique rules for how the child can walk on them. For example, if the tape is blue, the kid has to walk with one hand on his head, or if it is green, he has to limp the stretch.
- The child has to follow the rules and walk only on the tape and not on open land! If he does, he's out.
- The child who walks the length of the tape without

stepping on the bare floor wins.

Quick Tip:

You can make different variations of this game by using
multiple colored masking tapes and creating different
patterns. You can also make it more interesting by making the
child walk backward.

Listening game

This game is both educational and fun for younger kids. The game exercises the child's listening abilities by compelling them to concentrate.

You will need:

- A lot of miscellaneous items that have a distinct sound

How to:

- Collect items such as combs, vessels, remote, books, pens, bottles, toys, clocks, etc., which have unique sounds.
- Place the items on the table and ask the child to make a mental note of them.
- Take the items away and ask the kid to turn the other side or close his eyes.
- Pick an item and make a sound with it. If the child guesses it correctly, he scores a point.

Quick Tip:

You could use a blindfold to make sure the kid is not peeking!

Pitching pennies

Pitching pennies is a cool game to develop the child's hand-eye coordination. Similar to beer pong, the game is for the entire family.

You will need:

- Pennies or other small currency coins
- Plastic or paper drinking cups (large size)

How to:

- Each child gets five coins. A cup is placed on a table or a chair in front of them.
- Ask the child to take 'x' steps away from the cup, where 'x' is his or her age. Adults can move five steps farther than the children to throw the pennies.

- The child has to toss the coins, one at a time, into the cup.

- The child who puts in most coins in five chances wins.

Quick Tip:

You can replace coins with marbles or even ping pong balls.

In and out hangman

An excellent variation of the classic game, in and out can be used to revise lessons with kids.

You will need:

- White or black board

- Marker or chalk

- Set of questions and answers

How to:

- Ask the child a question and draw as many tiny blanks as there are letters in the answers. Use proper spacing to separate words and make it easier for the child to guess the answer.

- In the classic version, you guess the letters that are in the phrase or word. In this version, you alternate between letters that are in the words and letters that are not in it.

- So if the child guesses a letter that is 'in' the word or phrase in the first chance, then in the second chance, he should guess a letter that is 'not in' (or 'out') of the word or phrase.

- Every player is allowed seven wrong guesses or as many steps as it takes to draw the stick hangman figure.

Quick Tip:

Make the game fun by having quizzes about your child's favorite movie, TV show, or singer.

Pen and pencil games

There are a few pen and pencil games that you can play at home, on the plane, or in the car.

You will need:

- Plain sheet of paper
- Pencil
- Eraser

Games you can play:

- **Join the dots:** Make a 6×6 square of dots on a page. Take turns to join dots with a line. You can join only two dots at a time. If your line completes a box, you put your initial inside it. The person with the highest number of boxes wins. Once the child gets the hang of the game, move to a bigger square.
- **Tic Tac Toe** is another game you can play using a pencil and paper. The game is played on a 3×3 grid square. The first person puts an 'X' in one of the grids and the second player puts an 'O'. The first player to

successfully get three Xs or Os in a line (vertical, horizontal, or diagonal) wins. You can also play this using a whiteboard and marker.

- **Pictionary** is similar to charades. However, the person who has to express word or phrase needs to draw instead of acting it out.

- **Name, place, animal, thing:** Divide the page into four parts: Name, Place, Animal, Thing. Set a timer for a few seconds and let the child recite the alphabet silently. When the timer stops, the child says what letter he stopped at, and the players have to write down the names of a person, animal, thing, and place starting with that letter.

Sock toss

This is like basketball inside the house, except you use socks instead of a ball and clothes hamper instead of the basket.

You will need:

- A bunch of colorful socks
- A bucket or clothes hamper
- Space to play

How to:

- Roll up the socks into tiny balls and tie them up.
- Place the clothes basket a few feet away from where you are standing.
- Take turns to throw the socks into the basket.
- Move one step back each time you get the sock into the basket.

Quick Tip:

You could make this a little difficult for older kids by choosing a basket or bin with a smaller opening.

Indoor obstacle course

Indoor obstacle courses need space. If you have a big house with enough space and the house has child-proofed areas, you must try this on a snowy or rainy day.

You will need:

- Hula hoops

- Chairs

- Blankets

- Exercise ball

- You can add anything else that might be useful.

How to:

- Create an obstacle course with specific rules on what to do or how to maneuver around each obstacle.

- For example, if there is a chair or a table, tell the kids that they have to crawl under it. If there is a hula hoop, they have to use the hoop twice or thrice before moving on to the next obstacle and so on.

- The child gets a score only if he or she has passed all the obstacles as they should have.

Puzzles

When you cannot step out, pick up a few puzzles that you can work on all day.

You will need:

A lot of puzzles games, books, and ideas

Types of puzzles:

- **Picture puzzles**, but these won't keep you busy for long unless there are more than 25 pieces in it.

- A **picture puzzle** book can be a great idea, given that you can work on one puzzle after another to keep the child engaged.

- **Word puzzles** are a great option if you want to improve your child's vocabulary.

- **3D puzzles** toys are good for younger children.

Quick Tip:

Stock up a few puzzle books or games in the house, without your child's knowledge, to save yourself on a rainy day.

Card games

Kids can play card games too. Pick simple games that can help improve the child's logical reasoning, number identification, and arrangement and color segregation abilities.

You will need:

- A deck or two of cards

Card games you can play:

Popular kids' card games you can play include:

- **Spoons**, which is good for three players or more

- **Garbage or trash**, which is for two players

- Card **memory game** is similar to Mahjong. You will need two sets of a suit from two decks of cards.

- **Go Fish**, which is great for preschoolers and younger kids

- **Crazy Eights**, where the objective is to get rid of all cards

- **Pounce**, a fast-paced card game for two people

Build a fort

You won't need any boulders or cement to build a fort indoors. Gather a few things from around the house, and you are all set.

You will need:

What you need depends on the type of fort you want to build: Pillows, blankets, sticks, cardboard boxes, and furniture such as chairs or tables.

Types of forts:

- Cardboard forts are perhaps the easiest to build if you

have boxes of the right size. Gather a few large boxes
and join them using tape. Build it any way you want, but
in such a way that your kid can sit or sleep comfortably
in it.

- Pillow forts are perhaps the most popular among
children, for they are soft and fun to make. You will,
however, need a lot of different types of pillows for this.
You can also use stacks of blankets and towels and some
sturdy furniture to hold the fort.

- Teepee tents are the simplest DIY indoor conical tents
that can be made with a sheet of cloth and a few sticks.

-

- Blanket and furniture fort is what you can create in a
short time. Just empty a table and cover it completely
with a large blanket or bed sheet. Fold the blanket up in
the front to indicate the opening or entrance to the fort.

Quick Tip:

You could also make a combination fort with pillows,
blankets, and cardboard boxes.

Dominoes

Stacking up the dominoes and then watching them fall one by one is just something! And that is exactly what you should do when you have all day to yourself.

You will need:

- Dominoes game set

How to:

- Stack up the dominoes in any pattern you like. Get your child to help you with the design and arrangement. This may take you a couple of hours or so, depending on the number of dominoes in the set.

- Once it is ready, you can ask your child to flip the first domino to set it off while you can record on video!

Quick Tip:

Come up with different patterns and time them to see which takes the longest to fall.

Marshmallow tinker toys

Marshmallows are not just for eating. They can also be used, with pretzels, to make tinker toys.

You will need:

- A bag of marshmallows
- A bag or two of pretzels

How to:

- Break the pretzels into sticks that can be used to join two marshmallows.
- Join the marshmallows to create a house, car, soldier, snowman, or anything else.

Quick Tip:

Let the child create anything he or she wants to with the marshmallows. Let the child's imagination soar with this activity.

Make your own story

Another way to boost your child's creative abilities is to make them tell you a story.

You will need:

- A few ideas for storytelling

How to:

- If you have older kids, pick a theme and ask them to tell you a story.
- With younger kids, start a story and ask them to continue it midway. That will give them some footing and also ideas for a plot.

Quick Tip:

Your kid's stories may not always make sense. But don't stop them or correct them. Let them weave the story as they want. After all, it is fiction and need not be true.

Sometimes, children's stories could be things that have actually happened to them. Read between the lines and talk to them if necessary, to figure out if it is just their imagination or reality.

DIY catapult

This is a fun activity but needs time and patience. The thrill is in making your own catapult and then using it to toss marshmallows.

You will need:

- Popsicle sticks
- Elastic rubber bands
- A plastic spoon

How to:

- Stack up five popsicle sticks and bind them on both ends using a rubber band. Make four more Popsicle sticks with four sticks each.
- Place one stack horizontally and three perpendicularly, and bind them to the horizontal one using more rubber

bands.

- Tie the plastic spoon to the other popsicle stack, place it
  vertically on the other side of the larger stack (horizontal
  stack), and secure it using bands.

- The catapult is now ready for play. Place a marshmallow
  in the spoon and try to toss it into another person's
  mouth or a cup.

Ice tower excavation

Ice tower excavation is a cool game that your children will
enjoy during summers when it is too hot to go outside.

You will need:

- A long/tall container

- Colorful trinkets like beads, shapes, marbles, etc.

How to:

- Fill the container with clear water and drop the toys in
  it.

- Put the bottle in the freezer, until the water turns into a block of ice.

- Ease the ice tower out of the bottle and give the child squeeze bottles, salt, and eye droppers as tools to melt the ice and rescue the trinkets.

Quick Tip:

Pick a container which is uniform, throughout, in width. That way, getting the ice tower out of the container becomes easier.